An Introduction to CBD Oil:

Promote your Health and Well-being, Treat Anxiety, Pain, Autism and More, All Naturally

By

Jana Ceesay

Table Of Contents

Introduction

CBD stands for cannabidiol oil. It is used to treat different symptoms even though its use is rather controversial. There is also some confusion and controversy as to how exactly the oil affects our bodies. Cannabidiol oil and other cannabis derived products may have significant health benefits and are legal in many places today.

CBD is a cannabinoid, a compound found in cannabis plant, also known as marijuana. The oil contains CBD concentrations and the uses vary greatly. In cannabis, the compound that is well known for its rather mind-altering properties is "delta 9 tetrahydrocannabinol," or THC. It is an active ingredient found in marijuana. Marijuana has both CBD and THC, and each has different effects.

THC alters the mind when one is smoking or cooking with it. This is because it is broken down by heat. Unlike THC, CBD isn't psychoactive. This means that your state of mind does not change with its use. However, significant changes can be noted within the human body, suggesting medical benefits.

The term "CBD" is a nickname for cannabidiol, which is one of several cannabinoids, or chemical compounds, that are found in cannabis and hemp plants. Of course, the most famous cannabinoid is tetrahydrocannabinol, or THC, which is the main psychoactive component in marijuana (aka, the part that gets you high). Because CBD is not psychoactive, it does not create the same buzzy effects typically associated with marijuana when ingested. But just because CBD won't get you high, that doesn't mean it has no side effects or potential uses.

What does it do?

Because of the overall legal ambiguity around the cannabis plant (marijuana is federally illegal, but dozens of states have legalized it for medical and/or recreational purposes in recent years), the jury is still out, somewhat, when it comes to the potential benefits and medical applications of cannabidiol.

Still, CBD is already commonly used to relieve some symptoms of anxiety, including insomnia, and there have been some studies that show it to be effective in those cases. Other studies have shown that CBD could have anti-inflammatory properties, and many CBD products are marketed for relieving chronic pain, such as arthritis. And multiple studies have found CBD to be an effective treatment for seizures, and there are various CBD products that are used by patients with epilepsy. However, major health agencies like the U.S. Food and Drug Administration, National Institutes of Health and the

World Health Organization have all stated in recent years that additional CBD testing and research is necessary.

Chapter One

How do you use it?

Once the CBD compound is extracted from cannabis and hemp plants, it is typically packaged in the form of concentrated oil or cream. For trendy wellness products, the oil is mixed or infused in any number of other goods, including pills, vaporizers, beauty creams, shampoos and edibles like candy, mints and flavored sparkling water. You can even get CBD-infused pet treats that are marketed to owners of dogs and cats suffering from anxiety.

And there's a growing culture of CBD cocktail enthusiasts, spurred on by the likes of Food & Wine magazine and Gwyneth Paltrow's growing health and wellness empire, Goop. For medicinal purposes, creams and balms that claim to treat pain can be rubbed directly on the skin and CBD oils can be taken orally, often with a dropper that deposits a drop or two in your mouth.

Is it safe?

Again, the more studies and medical research that focus on CBD, the more will be known about its side effects and potential medical benefits. For what it's worth, in December 2017, the World Health Organization declared in a report that "cannabidiol does not appear to have abuse potential or cause harm." The WHO also noted that CBD could have "therapeutic value" for epileptic seizures, but that further study is warranted to determine CBD's potential medical use.

Then, in June, the FDA approved GW Pharmaceutical's Epidiolex, a CBD-based drug for treating epileptic seizures — marking the first time the agency has ever approved a drug derived from marijuana.

However, it's also worth noting that there have been several instances where the FDA has issued warnings to companies for illegally marketing CBD products with overblown and unrealistic claims, including that they can cure cancer.

But, is it legal?

Well, much like with other cannabis products, that's kind of a gray area. On the federal level, any CBD products derived from cannabis plants are completely illegal, unless they are approved by the FDA (which only includes Epidiolex at the moment), the Drug Enforcement Agency said in September. The DEA even told VICE recently that the federal law makes no distinction between CBD derived from cannabis or hemp (a cannabis plant species with an especially low concentration of THC grown legally in roughly 40 states, mostly for industrial purposes). In other words, the official stance of the federal government seems to be that CBD products are illegal whether they are derived from cannabis or hemp.

However (and this is very important), as has typically been the case with legal marijuana, the federal government mostly looks the other way while individual states decide how to treat CBD. As such, most states allow CBD products in some form, usually for medical purposes. The 30 states that have legalized medical marijuana include CBD products in that protection, while a number of other states have specific CBD laws that allow for those products in some form, so long as they also contain no more than a miniscule amount of THC. Only four states consider all cannabis-derived products, including CBD, to be illegal: Idaho, South Dakota, Nebraska and Kansas.

Meanwhile, CBD derived solely from hemp could soon be legal everywhere. Senate Majority Leader Mitch McConnell is backing a new legislation that would remove hemp from the DEA's list of controlled substances, which would make it legal across the country (along with products made from hemp).

In short, CBD's legal status in the U.S. may still not be entirely clear, but with the potential for billions of dollars in sales in the coming years, it doesn't seem to be going away anytime soon.

How CBD Oil works

Cannabinoids affect the body by attaching themselves to different receptors. Some cannabinoids are produced by the body and there are the CB1 and CB2 receptors. CB1 receptors are located all through the body with a great number of them being in the brain. The receptors are responsible for mood, emotions, pain, movement, coordination, memories, appetite, thinking, and many other functions. THC affects these receptors.

As for the CB2 receptors, they are mainly in one's immune system and affect pain and inflammation. Even though CBD does not attach directly here, it directs the body to use cannabinoids more.

 CBD is beneficial to human health in different ways. It is a natural pain reliever and has anti-inflammatory properties. Over the counter drugs are used for pain relief and most people prefer a more natural alternative and this is where CBD oil comes in.

Research has shown that CBD provides a better treatment, especially for people with chronic pain.

There is also evidence that suggest that the use of CBD can be very helpful for anyone who is trying to quit smoking and dealing with drug withdrawals. In a study, it was seen that smokers who had inhalers that had CBD tended to smoke less than what was usual for them and without any further craving for cigarettes. CBD could be a great treatment for persons with addiction disorders especially to opioids.

There are many other medical conditions that are aided by CBD and they include epilepsy, LGA, Dravet syndrome, seizures and so on. More research is being conducted on the effects of CBD in the human body and the results are quite promising. The possibility of combating cancer and different anxiety disorders is also being looked at.

Chapter Two

Things Everyone Gets Wrong About CBD

The past year has seen a surge of interest in marijuana's CBD, a non-intoxicating cannabis compound with significant therapeutic properties. Numerous commercial start-ups and internet retailers have jumped on the CBD bandwagon, touting CBD derived from industrial hemp as the next big thing, a miracle oil that can shrink tumors, quell seizures, and ease chronic pain — without making people feel "stoned." But along with a growing awareness of cannabidiol as a potential health aid, there has been a proliferation of misconceptions about CBD.

Project CBD receives many inquiries from around the world and oftentimes people say they are seeking "CBD, the medical part" of the plant, "not THC, the recreational part" that gets you high. Actually, THC, "The High Causer," has awesome therapeutic properties. Scientists at the Scripps Research Center in San Diego reported that THC inhibits an enzyme implicated in the formation of beta-amyloid plaque, the hallmark of Alzheimer's-related dementia.

The federal government recognizes single-molecule THC (Marinol) as an anti-nausea compound and appetite booster, deeming it a Schedule III drug, a category reserved for medicinal substances with little abuse potential. But whole plant marijuana, the only natural source of THC, continues to be classified as a dangerous Schedule I drug with no medical value.

- ### THC is the "bad" cannabinoid. CBD is the good cannabinoid

The drug warrior's strategic retreat: Give ground on CBD while continuing to demonize THC. Diehard marijuana prohibitionists are exploiting the good news about CBD to further stigmatize high-THC cannabis, casting tetrahydrocannabinol as the bad cannabinoid, whereas CBD is framed as the good cannabinoid. Why? Because CBD doesn't make you high like THC does.

- ### CBD is most effective without THC

THC and CBD are the power couple of cannabis compounds — they work best together. Scientific studies have established that CBD and THC interact synergistically to enhance each other's therapeutic effects. British researchers have shown that CBD potentiates THC's anti-inflammatory properties in an animal model of colitis.

Scientists at the California Pacific Medical Center in San Francisco determined that a combination of CBD and THC has a more potent anti-tumoral effect than either compound alone when tested on brain cancer and breast cancer cell lines. And extensive clinical research has demonstrated that CBD combined with THC is more beneficial for neuropathic pain than either compound as a single molecule.

- **Single-molecule pharmaceuticals are superior to 'crude' whole-plant medicinals**

According to the federal government, specific components of the marijuana plant (THC, CBD) have medical value, but the plant itself does not have medical value. Uncle Sam's single-molecule blinders reflect a cultural and political bias that privileges Big Pharma products. Single-molecule medicine is the predominant corporate way, the FDA-approved way, but it's not the only way, and it's not necessarily the optimal way to benefit from cannabis therapeutics.

- **CBD is CBD, it doesn't matter where it comes from**

Yes, it does matter. The flower-tops and leaves of some industrial hemp strains may be a viable source of CBD (legal issues notwithstanding), but hemp is by no means an optimal source of cannabidiol. Industrial hemp typically contains far less cannabidiol than CBD-rich cannabis. Huge amounts of industrial hemp are required to extract a small amount of CBD, thereby raising the risk of toxic contaminants because hemp is a "bio-accumulator" that draws heavy metals from the soil. Single-molecule CBD synthesized in a lab or extracted and refined from industrial hemp lacks critical medicinal terpenes and secondary cannabinoids found in cannabis strains. These compounds interact with CBD and THC to enhance their therapeutic benefits.

Everything you need to know about CBD oil

People take or apply cannabidiol to treat a variety of symptoms, but its use is controversial. There is some confusion about what it is and how it affects the human body.

Cannabidiol (CBD) may have some health benefits, and it may also pose risks. Products containing the compound are now legal in many American states where marijuana is not. This chapter will explain what you don't know about CBD oil, its possible health benefits, how to use it, potential risks.

- **Is CBD marijuana?**

Until recently, the best-known compound in cannabis was delta-9 tetrahydrocannabinol (THC). This is the most active ingredient in marijuana. Marijuana contains both THC and CBD, and these compounds have different effects. THC creates a mind-altering "high" when a person smokes it or uses it in cooking. This is because THC breaks down when we apply heat and introduce it into the body.

CBD is different. Unlike THC, it is not psychoactive. This means that CBD does not change a person's state of mind when they use it. However, CBD does appear to produce significant changes in the body, and some research suggests that it has medical benefits.

- **Where does CBD come from?**

The least processed form of the cannabis plant is hemp. Hemp contains most of the CBD that people use medicinally. Hemp and marijuana come from the same plant, Cannabis sativa, but the two are very different. Over the years, marijuana farmers have selectively bred their plants to contain high levels of THC and other compounds that interested them, often because the compounds produced a smell or had another effect on the plant's flowers. However, hemp farmers have rarely modified the plant. These hemp plants are used to create CBD oil.

- **How CBD works**

All cannabinoids, including CBD, produce effects in the body by attaching to certain receptors. The human body produces certain cannabinoids on its own. It also has two receptors for cannabinoids, called the CB1 receptors and CB2 receptors. CB1 receptors are present throughout the body, but many are in the brain. The CB1 receptors in the brain deal with coordination and movement, pain, emotions, and mood, thinking, appetite, and memories, and other functions. THC attaches to these receptors. CB2 receptors are more common in the immune system. They affect inflammation and pain. Researchers once believed that CBD attached to these CB2 receptors, but it now appears that CBD does not attach directly to either receptor. Instead, it seems to direct the body to use more of its own cannabinoids.

Chapter Three

Cannabis Oil Vs. Smoking Marijuana

When people picture the words marijuana or cannabis, they often conjure images of getting high. Those images are terribly wrong when cannabis oil is substituted for rolled marijuana joints. Taking cannabis oil and smoking marijuana can both yield health benefits, but both are also too different in several ways.

- **Medicinal Benefits**

Both using cannabis oil and smoking marijuana yield different medical benefits. Smoking cannabis has been useful in treating diseases like glaucoma and nausea. It can be used to alleviate chronic pain and may even help reduce the size or stop the growth of cancer, as well as stop the progression of Alzheimer's disease. Cannabis oil is also used to treat cancer and nausea, but it can also improve sleep, protect the skin, combat stress and anxiety and promote heart health. Both may be used to treat symptoms of post-traumatic stress disorder (PTSD), headaches and migraines. They may also be used to combat the symptoms of multiple sclerosis and premenstrual syndrome. Typically, the oil contains concentrated cannabinoid profiles for more potency, but many primarily include cannabidiol (CBD), which does not get people high. For this reason, some states allow children to take advantage of CBD oils for certain illnesses and conditions.

- Legality

The legality of smoked cannabis and oils differs by state, with some allowing only one or the other. Likewise, some states only approved the plant for use in a limited capacity, such as for children with epileptic disorders. It continues to be classified as a Schedule I drug, making it illegal under federal stipulations. When produced from industrial hemp products, cannabis oil may be legal, but when created from a crop of medical marijuana, its status reverts back to illegal unless the state has provisions for it.

- Safety

Inhaling cannabis may involve minor issues due to the combustion process, while using cannabis oil does not result in the same effects since it does not require being heated. Since its benefits can be enjoyed without smoking, the remedy is often considered for children with severe health conditions, like epilepsy. Smokers may want to consider a vaporizer for whole-plant cannabis consumption.

Psychoactive Properties

Tetrahydrocannabinol (THC) is the naturally occurring compound that famously produces cannabis' mind-altering states. The CBD compound found in the plant, however, does not have psychoactive properties. CBD produces a calming effect on the mind, making it a good treatment for people with social anxiety and other nervous disorders. When combined with THC in stronger amounts, CBD can help balance out the medication, ensuring that the user does not get too high. Oil can be slightly harder to procure and more expensive than medical marijuana flowers, depending on state laws. Smoking cannabis can be more beneficial to some people, largely depending on their condition.

Does CBD Oil Really Work?

The popularity of medical marijuana is soaring, and among the numerous products consumers are seeking are cannabis oils — the most in-demand of which is referred to simply as CBD oil.

A wealth of marketing material, blogs and anecdotes claim that cannabis oils can cure whatever ails you, even cancer. But the limited research doesn't suggest that cannabis oil should take the place of conventional medication, except for in two very rare forms of epilepsy (and even then, it's recommended only as a last-resort treatment). And, experts caution that because cannabis oil and other cannabis-based products are not regulated or tested for safety by the government or any third-party agency, it's difficult for consumers to know exactly what they're getting.

How does CBD affect the body?

Marijuana and CBD work by acting on the body's endocannabinoid system. This system's main job is to maintain homeostasis and help the body adapt to outside stressors.

There are two main types of cannabinoids—endo (produced naturally within the body) and phyto (produced from a plant). CBD is one type of phytocannabinoid. Phytocannabinoids mimic endocannabinoids, so they can act like a supplement, giving you a boost beyond what your body can produce.

Receptors for cannabinoids are found in the digestive, reproductive, nervous, and immune systems. Because cannabinoids interact with almost every system in our bodies, they're often touted as a cure-all. While they're not truly able to heal everything, they do regulate neurotransmitter function, inflammation, mitochondrial function, and metabolism.

Who should try CBD oil?

CBD is safe for almost everyone, according to a recent report from the World Health Organization, but check with your doctor before starting any CBD product, especially if you are pregnant or on any medications. Research has shown several CBD oil benefits, ranging from alleviating social anxiety to improving rheumatoid arthritis.

CBD health benefits.

Improves mood disorders.

CBD works directly on the brain receptors 5HT1A (serotonin) and GABA (an inhibitory neurotransmitter). Lower levels of these can contribute to anxiety and depression.

Lowers inflammation.

Suppresses cytokine production and induces T-regulatory cells to protect the body from attacking itself, which can help autoimmune conditions.

Decreases chronic pain.

Inhibits transmission of neuronal signalling through pain pathways.

Aids gut health.

Helps heal the leaky tight junctions that contribute to intestinal permeability and decreases spasmodic activity common in irritable bowel syndrome.

Helps treat seizures.

May relieve epilepsy in children.

Does CBD Oil Create a High?

The short answer is: No. (Though oils with THC can also contain CBD). There are two different types of CBD oil products — hemp-based CBD oil (the one I'm talking about in this article) and marijuana-based CBD (which is what someone would buy at the dispensary). Both contain CBD, and they're both derived from the cannabis plant, but hemp and medical marijuana are are different varieties of the plant.

Marijuana-based CBD is generally going to have more THC and other cannabinoids. CBD oil does not contain THC (the compound that causes a "high" feeling). This is an important distinction that many people don't understand.

The variety that is typically (and legally) used to make CBD oil is hemp. How is hemp oil different? A plant can only be legally considered hemp if it contains .3% per dry unit (or less) of the compound THC.

In a nutshell, CBD oil or hemp oil contains the benefits of the cannabis plant without the potential drawbacks of psychoactive compounds typically found from inhalation or other methods of consumption.

Chapter Four

Cannabidiol (CBD) Uses for Pain, Inflammation & Epilepsy

CBD oil is a great remedy for a lot of different ailments. Here are some of the amazing uses people (and medical research) report for CBD oil:

1. Relief for Chronic Pain

Those suffering from chronic pain from diseases like fibromyalgia are finding relief with CBD. Taking CBD can offer pain relief and can even prevent nervous system degeneration. In fact, it has been approved in Canada for multiple sclerosis and cancer pain.

What's really amazing is that CBD doesn't cause dependence or tolerance, so it's a great choice for those trying to stay away from opioids.

Other Remedies to Consider: Not into CBD? Research also shows that turmeric consumption and heat therapy (like sauna use) may be helpful as well. A low inflammation diet also seems to be helpful for some people.

2. Calms Childhood Epilepsy

CBD has anti-seizure properties that have been shown to successfully treat drug-resistant children who have neurological disorders like epilepsy (with no side effects!). In one study published in the New England Journal of Medicine, CBD decreased frequency of seizures by 23 percentage points more than those taking a placebo.

Other Remedies to Consider: Childhood epilepsy is a serious condition and it is important to work with a ualified practitioner with a specialty in this area. Emerging research also shows that a ketogenic diet can be very helpful for drug resistant epilepsy, especially in children.

3. Reduces Anxiety and Depression

According to the Anxiety and Depression Association of America, depression affects 6% and anxiety affects 18% of the U.S. population each year. Research shows that CBD oil can help with both.

CBD has been shown to reduce levels of stress and anxiety in those suffering from conditions such as PTSD, social anxiety disorder, and obsessive compulsive disorder. CBD even reduced the stress and discomfort surrounding public speaking.

Though a B12 deficiency may also be to blame, CBD has been shown to reduce depression by enhancing both serotonergic and glutamate cortical signaling (both are lacking in those with depression). Other Remedies to Consider: Dr Kelly Brogan provides a lot of helpful information for anxiety and depression in this podcast episode. Vitamin B12 is also linked to mental health and it may be helpful to work with someone experienced in optimizing levels of B12.

4. Fights Multi-Drug Resistant Bacteria

Researchers discovered that cannabinoids (including CBD) have an unusual ability to destroy bacteria (especially drug-resistant strains). More research is needed to find out how and why it works. CBD can also slow the progression of tuberculosis in rats. Researchers concluded that CBD likely does this by inhibiting T-cell proliferation, rather than possessing antibacterial properties. Whatever the mechanism is for destroying bacteria, CBD seems to be a potent weapon against the antibiotic resistant "superbugs" that are becoming more and more of a problem today.

Other Remedies to Consider: Don't want to try cannabidiol? There is also research on using garlic, honey and oregano oil for drug resistant strains, but work with a practitioner experienced in infectious disease.

5. Reduces Inflammation

Chronic inflammation is a huge problem in our society that contributes to many non-infectious diseases including heart disease, cancer, Alzheimer's, autoimmune disease, and more, according to the National Center for Biotechnology Information.

Diet and lifestyle play a huge part in chronic inflammation but when folks are already eating a healthy, nutrient-dense diet and optimizing their lifestyle (getting enough sleep and exercise for example), CBD oil can help. Research also shows that CBD oil can reduce chronic inflammation that leads to disease.

Other Remedies to Consider: Research agrees that it is important to address gut health to manage inflammation. Removing refined sugar from the diet has also been shown to reduce inflammation in as little as a week.

6. Reduces Oxidative Stress

Oxidative stress is responsible for many ailments today. Oxidative stress is when the body has too many free radicals and can't keep up with neutralizing them (with antioxidants). This is more of a problem now than in the past because our environment is so much more toxic than it once was. A 2010 study shows that CBD oil acts as an antioxidant and another study found CBD has neuroprotective qualities. So CBD can reduce neurological damage caused by free radicals.

7. Help for Schizophrenia

Schizophrenia is a complicated and serious disease that is typically managed through therapy and pharmaceutical drugs (that carry hefty side effects). Anecdotally, many folks have found that CBD oil has helped reduce hallucinations. Research is beginning to catch up too. A March 2015 review of available research found that CBD was a safe, effective, and well tolerated treatment for psychosis. But more research is needed to bring CBD into clinical practice. It should be mentioned that THC, the psychoactive compound in marijuana, may actually increase psychosis for those at risk. CBD oil, on the other hand, only helps reduce psychosis and may even counteract psychosis brought on by marijuana use.

8. Promotes Healthy Weight

Cannabidiol can help maintain healthy blood sugar, stimulates genes and proteins that helps break down fat, and increase mitochondria that helps burn calories. CBD also encourages the body to convert white fat to brown fat. White fat is the kind of fat we typically think of when we think about body fat. Brown fat is fat that is in small deposits that behaves differently than white fat. Brown fat is said to improve health by enhancing the bodies ability to burn white fat, create heat, and even regulate blood sugar.

9. Improves Heart Health

Heart disease is a growing problem today. In fact, it's the leading cause of death in the U.S. A healthy diet and lifestyle is a top priority for heart health, but CBD oil can also help. According to research cannabidiol reduces artery blockage, reduces stress induced cardiovascular response, and can reduce blood pressure. It may also reduce cholesterol.

As mentioned earlier, CBD oil is helpful in preventing oxidative stress and inflammation. Both of these are often precursors to heart disease.

10. Improves Skin Conditions

CBD oil can be used topically to treat skin conditions. Studies show CBD oil has a high potential for treating skin conditions like eczema by encouraging abnormal cell death. It can also help regulate the skin's oil production, reducing acne. CBD also contains many nutrients like vitamin E that help improve and protect the skin.

Other Remedies to Consider: Diet is vitally important for skin health. Many people find that removing foods like sugar, dairy or grains (if sensitive) improves skin. I also personally use a skin probiotic spray that has made a huge difference for my acne prone skin.

11. Fights Cancer

CBD oil's role in cancer treatment still needs more research, but what is available is looking promising. According to the American Cancer Society, CBD oil can slow growth and spread of some kinds of cancer (in animals). Because it fights oxidative stress and inflammation (and both are linked to cancer) it makes sense that CBD oil could help fight cancer cells.

Chapter Five

CBD vs. Hemp Oil

This is a common ⬜uestion and misconception. As mentioned above, while they come from the same plant, they are different strains and CBD is harvested from the plants that contain no THC (or negligible levels). CBD is completely legal and is not considered a drug. Because of the often confused history of these plants, many manufacturers use "hemp oil" instead of the more controversial "CBD oil" in their marketing. CBD levels can vary drastically based on manufacturing, so it is important to find a high quality manufacturer with verified levels.

From a sustainability standpoint, it is a shame that hemp has gotten so much negative press because it comes from a similar strain of plant. Aside from the CBD benefits, hemp is one of the strongest, longest, and most durable natural fibers and it can be grown without any type of pesticides or herbicides! It also:

- makes up to four times as much fiber per acre as pine trees
- can be recycled many more times than pine-based pulp products
- is easy to grow without chemicals and is actually good for the soil
- produces a seed and seed oil rich in protein, essential fatty acids and amino acids

CBD oil is most often used internally (through ingestion). Because CBD oil is a relatively new supplement, exact dosing isn't well established. While more long-term studies are needed, there is no established CBD "overdose" and there are very few if any side effects at any dosage.

When trying to find the right dosage, consider these things:

- Start by purchasing a high quality oil from a reputable company. A higher ⬜uality oil will be more bioavailable, so a lower dose can be enough.
- Begin with the recommended dosage on the bottle (especially if using preventatively).
- Some notice a change immediately, while others don't notice any improvement for several weeks. If after several weeks there is still no change, increase the dosage.
- As with most herbal supplements, a small dosage 3-4 times a day is usually more therapeutic than one large dose.

Important note: Though CBD oil on its own is very safe, it may interact with medications, particularly opioids. Speak with your doctor if you're concerned about interactions or are unsure about using hemp oil for your conditions.

CBD Oil for Pets

Sidenote for our furrier friends: All mammals have an endocannabinoid system, CBD oil can have some of the same benefits for pets as it does for humans.

For cats and dogs in particular, CBD oil may help with:

- excessive barking or crying
- pets getting along with other pets
- pain
- relaxing pets before a trip to the vet
- lack of appetite
- separation anxiety

How to Use CBD Oil for Pets

There may be some trial and error in finding the right dosage for pets. Start with a low dose of 1 milligrams per 10 pounds of body weight and go up to 5 milligrams per 10 pounds of body weight if needed. A higher dose may be necessary for some ailments. A low dose 3-4 times a day is usually more therapeutic than one large dose.

Chapter Six

How CBD Oil Work with Autism

What is Autism?

Autism Spectrum Disorder (ASD) is a general condition of a brain development disorder. The disorders are characterized by difficulties in social communication and repetitive behaviors, besides being associated with intellectual disability, difficulties in coordination and attention, in some cases, hyperactivity, dyslexia, dyspraxia, anxiety, and depression.

Why CBD Oil to Treat Autism?

You might wonder why would researchers choose cannabis to treat Autism Spectrum Disorder?"

We know from the research that CBD can be used to effectively treat anxiety. CBD is one of the main cannabinoid compounds in cannabis. Unlike THC (tetrahydrocannabinol), the other main cannabinoid in cannabis, CBD is not psychoactive and has anti-anxiety properties. However, when it comes to cannabis or CBD, there are no published studies looking at the effect on ASD and its associated symptoms.

Despite the lack of clinical data, several lines of evidence led researchers to take a look at CBD-rich cannabis as a possible treatment of autism.

There is also an intriguing link between the endocannabinoid system — the neurotransmitter and receptor system in our bodies that is stimulated by cannabis-based cannabinoids like CBD and THC — and autism. According to a 2018 study published in Molecular Autism, children with ASD have lower concentrations of certain endocannabinoids in their blood. Administering CBD has also been effective at reducing the autistic-like social deficits in animal models of epilepsy and ASD.

A large proportion of children living with ASD also have socially disruptive behavioral problems such as tantrums, violence, and self-injury. Children with these severe symptoms are difficult to care for and often do not respond well to standard medical treatments. This has led caregivers to consider alternative therapies including medical cannabis.

Will CBD Be Used to Treat Autism?

This matter will re□uire many more studies, but the results of this study appear to validate the anecdotal evidence that CBD oil can help treat the symptoms of those living with Autism.

Overall, the researchers found positive changes in behavioral symptoms, communication problems, and levels of anxiety. 61% of the children's caregivers reporting "much improved" or "very much improved" symptoms.

The participants continued taking other medications during the study, including antipsychotics and mood stabilizers. However, many were able to take fewer medications, lower their dosages, or stop taking additional medications completely.

It's important to note that while the majority of the children who participated in the study showed improved behavior, 16 did not finish the study due to non-response, worsening symptoms, and in one case a psychotic episode.

How Does CBD Work With Autism?

From the moment that you start using a product that contains cannabidiol, whether it is edible or inhaled, you allow this compound to enter your body, into your bloodstream, and into your brain. As soon as it arrives, the cannabidiol interacts with specific receptors on the neurons called cannabinoids receptors, found in the cannabinoid systems that are spread throughout several areas of our nervous system.

Can CBD Help?

There is still no concrete scientific evidence to prove that CBD is an effective treatment for autism or epilepsy, therefore, many people are skeptical of the process and the ethics behind it. Fortunately, many researchers are conducting research trials to discover advanced science to back the CBD claims:

- *Cannabidiol Based Medical Cannabis in Children with Autism- A Retrospective Feasibility Study*

This retrospective study assessed the safety, tolerability, and efficacy of cannabidiol (CBD) based medical cannabis, as an adjuvant therapy, for refractory behavioral problems in children with ASD. Following the cannabis treatment, behavioral outbreaks were much improved or very much improved in 61% of patients. The anxiety and communication problems were much or very much improved by 39% and 47% respectively. Disruptive behaviors were improved by 29% following the treatment. Parents reported less stress as reflected in the APSI (Autism Parenting Stress Index) scores, changing by 33%. The effect on all outcome measures was more apparent in boys with non-syndromic ASD. Adverse events included sleep disturbances (14%) irritability (9%) and loss of appetite (9%).

- *Study to Explore Whether Cannabis Compound Eases Severe Symptoms of Autism*

Considered the most promising study about the relationship between cannabis and autism, this project was kickstarted with a donation of $4.7 million to the Center for Medicinal Cannabis Research (CMCR) at the UC San Diego School of Medicine. (This is considered the largest private donation to date for medicinal cannabis research in the US)The goals of the study include whether cannabis treatment is safe, tolerable, and effective in children with autism. The scientists predict research using the CBD for treatment, the substance of the plant that does not cause psychoactive effects and is most suitable for medical purposes. In addition, they seek to conclude whether the CBD alters the chemical messengers known as neurotransmitters, and how this process occurs, whether it is capable of improving brain connectivity and whether there is any change in biomarkers of brain inflammation, a symptom also associated with autism.

Conclusion

Hemp is a part of the cannabis plant and in most cases, it is not processed. This is where a lot of the CBD is extracted. Marijuana and hemp originate from cannabis sativa, but are ꓷuite different. Today, marijuana farmers are breeding plants so that they can have high THC levels. Hemp farmers do not need to modify plants and are used to create the CBD oil.

The wave of marijuana legalization in recent years has more and more Americans toking up legally and experimenting with everything from candy to skincare products infused with cannabis. But, there's one type of cannabis product that's been getting a lot of buzz — and, it won't even get you high.

CBD products have become increasingly popular in recent years, as more and more producers market CBD as the new "it" drug for the health and wellness set — one that has been touted as a pain reliever and a treatment for anxiety, among other potential applications. Last year, consumer sales of CBD products topped $350 million in the United states, more than triple the amount sold in 2014, and various estimates predict the market could reach $2 billion within the next two to four years.